# The B

## How to speed up healing of ligaments, tendons, and arthritis... naturally

### By

### Nathan Wei, MD, FACP, FACR

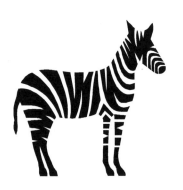

**www.arthritistreatmentcenter.com**

This book should not be a substitute for a thorough examination by your physician. The products that are mentioned in this book are recommended. Prior to using any of them, we recommend you seek advice from a qualified specialist. Neither the publisher nor the author may be held liable for any injury, loss, or damage sustained by anyone who relies on the information contained in the book.

# Table of Contents

# Introduction

Tissue regeneration- the ability to re-grow damaged tissues and organs has long been an elusive goal in medicine. Recent advances in the use of what are termed "bioactive" products, derived from a patient's own organs, have received much publicity.

Some of the information has, as a matter of course, been sensationalized. And there are a few medical practitioners who have touted themselves or been touted by the media as being authorities in the field.

The end result has been unreal expectations coupled with a sense of "faddism."

What is true and what is not?

This book serves to present the unvarnished facts. The information is derived from lengthy experience using both platelet-rich plasma, PRP, as well as stem cells in a busy research based arthritis center.

The material in this book has been distilled and translated from multiple scientific papers to make it both understandable as well as useful.

# Chapter 1

# What's New For Tendonitis? How About This… A Revolutionary Minimally Invasive Procedure That May Prevent Surgery!

Tendonitis refers to a condition where there is inflammation of a tendon or group of tendons. Tendons are the "ropes" that connect muscles to bones. Tendons can become irritated as a result of repetitive motion or trauma. What occurs is "overuse" which causes microtrauma or injury to the tendon. The fibers that make up the tendon begin to break down. This process is often accompanied by inflammation, particularly if there is underlying arthritis.

Tendons can also be inflamed where they insert into bone. Tendons are subject to irritation because they cross joints. When joints are used, so are tendons.

While repetitive motion is the usual culprit that leads to tendonitis, aging is also a factor.

Since tendons are ubiquitous – present at every joint in the body-tendonitis is a common malady. It most often occurs in the shoulder, elbow, wrist, hip, knee, and ankle.

The traditional approach to managing tendonitis has been to use non-steroidal anti-inflammatory drugs (NSAIDS) supplemented by rest, physical therapy, assistive devices such as splints, and corticosteroid injections.

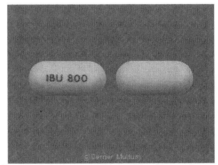

Anti-inflammatory drugs like ibuprofen are
often prescribed for tendonitis

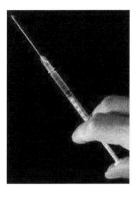

Glucocorticoid injections
("cortisone shots") are used to
alleviate pain with tendonitis

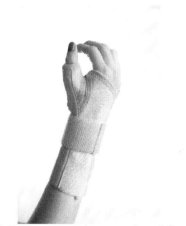

Splints are sometimes employed for
different types of tendonitis

In severe cases, open surgical procedures are performed.

Fortunately, there is a relatively new option that appears to be having surprisingly good results.

Since tendonitis is due to inflammation, the old thinking has been that reducing inflammation is the best approach. As a result, anti-inflammatory drugs, steroid injections, and so forth have been the mainstays of the "old school" of treatment.

Unfortunately, inflammation is also the body's attempt to heal the damage to the tendon. The problem is that inflammation is not always accompanied by the increased blood flow required to bring new nutrients to the area to help with the healing processes.

So, new techniques have been devised to actually try to temporarily increase blood flow through carefully and selectively injuring the tendon at the area of concern, and then stimulating the body's normal healing mechanisms to spring into action. While this seems paradoxical, it works.

The first part of this process involves the use of ultrasound guided percutaneous tenotomy (UGPT). Ultrasound is employed to aid in the diagnosis of the problem and then to guide the insertion of a needle to selectively injure the tendon at the site where tissue repair needs to occur.

The second part of the process is to inject a small amount of PRP (platelet-rich plasma). Platelets are small blood cells that are rich in various growth factors. These growth factors stimulate the growth and proliferation of new tissue. In essence, the platelet rich plasma helps regenerate new tendon fibers.

The procedure goes like this...

When the patient arrives at the clinic, the physician sits down and explains the procedure including risks and benefits.

The patients, if they agree to proceed, are taken to the laboratory and approximately 60 cc's of blood is drawn and then spun in a special centrifuge. After the specimen is spun, the layer containing platelets is drawn off using a special syringe.

The patient is first positioned in a comfortable manner on the procedure table.

The area of tendon pathology is then identified using diagnostic ultrasound. Often other problems that aggravate tendonitis such as bone spurs and arthritis will also be demonstrated.

After the informed consent is obtained, the area is sterilely prepared and anesthetized with a local anesthetic. A special needle of suitable gauge and length is inserted through the anesthetized skin and soft tissue and advanced to the tendon at the site of injury. Bone spurs, if present are gently chiseled away using the needle. Using carefully placed movements, multiple small holes are then placed in the tendon.

Since local anesthetic has been administered previously, a minimal amount of discomfort is experienced.

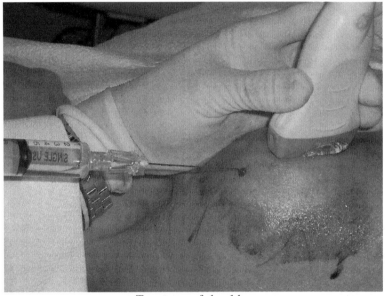
Tenotomy of shoulder

After the tendon has had multiple small holes placed – the needling procedure- a small amount of platelet-rich plasma (also called "autologous tissue grafting material") is slowly injected into the area.

The needle is then removed and a simple bandage is placed over the needle hole.

Post-procedure care consists of absolute rest for three days followed by modified rest for another four days, then slow and careful resumption of activity, along with physical therapy.

Analgesics such as tramadol (Ultram) or propoxyphene may be used. However, anti-inflammatory drugs and immunosuppressive drugs should be held for approximately a week before and a week after the treatment... and sometimes longer. The reason is we do not want anti-inflammatory effect to impede wound healing.

Ultrasound guided percutaneous tenotomy and autologous tissue grafting often prevents the need to perform an open surgical procedure. This outpatient procedure is done using either a regional block or local anesthetic.

A course of physical therapy may be initiated after the period of rest with the goals of improving function, decreasing pain, and increasing strength.

In some cases, a second course may be required. However, the long term results are extraordinary with very few patients requiring open surgery.

So who is a candidate for this procedure? Any patient with a history of chronic tendonitis that hasn't responded to other measures is a good candidate.

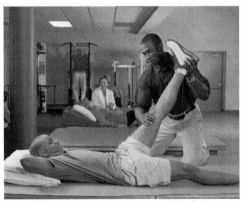
Physical therapy may be helpful

This includes people with arthritis who also have tendonitis (sometimes the distinction is not always easy to make and the arthritis pain may actually be tendon related pain). Patients with tendon rupture are not good candidates.

# Chapter 2

# Chronic Tendonitis... What's New in Treatment?

So, you've been diagnosed with tendonitis and you've gone through the usual types of treatment programs like physical therapy, anti-inflammatory drugs, and even cortisone shots.

What else is available?

Before we discuss the exciting new ways of managing chronic tendonitis, let's talk about what tendonitis is... and what it isn't.

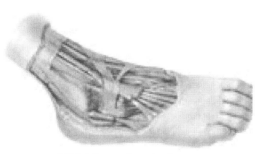

Multiple tendons in the front of the ankle.

Tendons are thick cords of fibrous tissue that connect muscles to bones. It is this connection that allows joint motion. When muscles contract, they pull on the tendons which cause the bones to move.

In order for tendons to glide they move inside a lubricated sheath of tissue that is lined with synovium. This synovial tissue is the same type of tissue that lines the inside of joints. Tendon pain can occur when the sheath through which a tendon glides becomes inflamed. Pain also occurs with degeneration or wear and tear of the tendon. This latter problem is the usual cause of tendon pain.

As a result, the term "tendonitis" should probably not be used. The correct term is actually "tendinosis." I will continue to use the term tendonitis though to keep things simple.

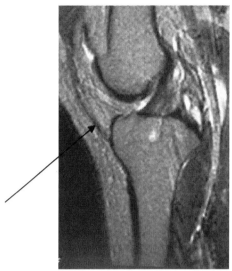

MRI study of patellar tendonitis

Tendon problems present with pain. The pain usually gets worse with use of the affected joint. However, when tendonitis becomes severe, there may be pain at rest, particularly at night.

Since muscles and tendons surround most joints, tendonitis is rather common. The diagnosis of tendonitis is relatively simple for the experienced clinician. Generally, the diagnosis is made by history and physical examination. In difficult diagnostic cases, diagnostic ultrasound or magnetic resonance imaging-MRI- is helpful in confirming the diagnosis.

Some of the more common types of tendonitis are:

First… shoulder tendonitis. The tendons in the shoulder that are most often affected are the rotator cuff and biceps tendons.

The rotator cuff consists of four tendons that sit on top of the upper arm bone. They are the supraspinatus, infraspinatus, subscapularis, and teres minor tendons. The location of these tendons and the muscles they attach to, are what give the shoulder such a great range of motion.

Rotator cuff tendonitis may occur as a result of repetitive activity or tendon degeneration. Pain is felt with most movements and is usually located on the outside part of the shoulder. Certain movements such as reaching behind or to the side may be uncomfortable.

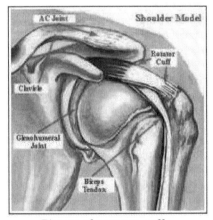

Picture of a rotator cuff

The biceps tendon permits the arm to be flexed at the elbow. Biceps tendonitis also occurs due to repetitive activity and pain is felt in the front of the shoulder.

Shoulder tendonitis can sometimes be treated successfully with anti-inflammatory medication, physical therapy, and occasionally glucocorticoid (cortisone) injection. These methods are most useful for acute tendonitis.

Tendonitis in the elbow is usually located on the outside and is called lateral epicondylitis or tennis elbow. It may also occur along the inside part of the elbow- medial epicondylitis. This is called golfer's elbow.

De Quervain's Tenosynovitis

Irritated tendons of the extensor pollicus brevis & abductor pollicus longus

www.arthritistreatmentcenter.com

## Lateral Epicondylitis

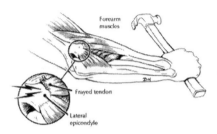

Treatment for these conditions consists of physical therapy, stretching and strengthening exercises, splints, and injections. While surgery is sometimes recommended for chronic cases, I will discuss why that is inadvisable.

Tendonitis in the wrist arises because of repetitive motion. A peculiar form of tendonitis, called DeQuervain's tendonitis, is felt on the outside of the thumb.

Tendonitis in this area is managed with glucorticoid injections and immobilization with a splint. Physical therapy modalities may be helpful. Rarely, if ever, is surgery required. Tendonitis in the fingers can lead to catching of the fingers. This is termed "trigger finger." Trigger finger usually responds to injection of glucocorticoid (cortisone).

Tendonitis in the hip is a complex problem. The hip joint is where the femur (leg bone) articulates with the pelvis. There is a bony prominence on the outside of the femur just below the joint, called the greater trochanter. This is a place where many tendons insert. It also is a place where tendonitis is common. Among the tendons in this location that can become inflamed on a common basis are the gluteus minimus, gluteus medius, pyriformis, obturator internus, gemelli, and quadratus femoris. Finding the exact site of pathology is important because if the exact location is not treated properly, the pain will continue.

Tendon and muscle problems in the front of the hip such as the sartorius, rectus femoris, iliacus, and adductor group can cause pain in the groin.

And in the back of the hip in the buttock region, tendonitis affecting the insertion of the semimembranosus, semitendonosus, and biceps femoris can also literally be a "pain in the butt."

Tendonitis in the knee may affect the patellar tendon. This is the tendon that connects the knee cap to the tibia (lower leg bone). Patellar tendonitis usually occurs because of excessive jumping and is actually called "jumpers knee." This is treated with rest, anti-inflammatory medications, and physical therapy.

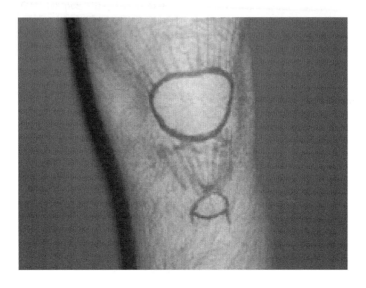

Patellar tendonitis. The area between the large oval (patella), and the small oval (tibial tubercle represents the Patellar tendon)

Tendonitis in the ankle can occur along the outside of the ankle (peroneal tendonitis), the inside of the ankle (posterior tibial tendonitis), or at the back of the ankle (Achilles tendonitis). The tendonitis that occurs along the outside or inside of the ankle can occur because of trauma or because of mechanical instability. Another potential cause is an underlying arthritis condition.

Achilles tendonitis often occurs as a result of excessive stress and loading of the tendon as well as repetitive motion. The Achilles tendon is the thick cord at the back of the ankle that connects the heel bone to the calf muscle. Treatment involves rest, elevation of the heel to take the tension off the Achilles tendon, and physical therapy. Glucocorticoid injection should be avoided because of the danger of causing Achilles tendon rupture. Anti-inflammatory medication may be helpful.

Achilles Tendon Illustrations

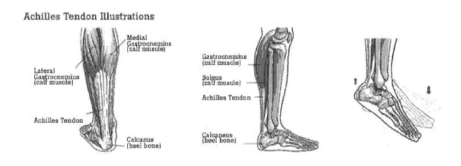

So what can be done to treat chronic tendonitis? What can you do if you've tried all of the above treatments and still have a problem?

The first new approach, particularly with tendons that are balky is to use hydrodissection. This is a form of treatment where a small gauge needle is introduced into the tendon sheath and a large volume of saline, glucocorticoid, and lidocaine are used to dissect the sheath away from the tendon. Often chronic inflammation causes the sheath and tendon to stick together and this can cause pain as well as loss of function. Hydrodissection is particularly effective for the small tendons in the hand.

Another new form of therapy called tenotomy is now being used. This almost always negates the need for an open surgical procedure. With tenotomy, a small gauge needle is introduced with local anesthetic and used to "irritate" the insertion of the tendon where the site of inflammation is located. The needle is inserted using direct ultrasound guidance and visualization. After the needling, injection of a small amount of platelet-rich plasma (PRP) is performed at the site of needling, again using direct ultrasound visualization. PRP is rich in growth factors that stimulate healing. The process of healing takes only a few days to weeks as opposed to the several weeks to months that an open surgical procedure takes.

Tenotomy can be performed at almost any site where there is chronic tendon inflammation. Results are usually excellent.

Sometimes the procedure may need to be repeated.

Both of these procedures are excellent for the aging athlete who wants to keep going.

# Chapter 3
# It All Starts With Wound Healing...

Wound healing is a complex process. It is characterized by:

- Multiple stages
- Complexity of interaction
- Participation by a wide variety of cells

The three stages of wound healing are:

- Inflammation
- Proliferation
- Remodeling

The first event that occurs after injury is hemostasis, meaning the formation of a clot. A clot consists of a mixture of platelets which contribute about 55 percent to clot strength and fibrin, which contributes about 45 percent to clot strength.

The second event is tissue regeneration.

To accelerate healing, there have been studies that demonstrate it is possible to initiate and accelerate tissue regeneration by using autologous (a patient's own) platelet concentrate. This concentrate is enriched with growth factors.

While the average platelet count in blood is about 200,000 per μl, the average platelet count in specially prepared platelet concentrates from plasma, PRP, is greater than 1,000,000. There is scientific proof of accelerated healing in bone and soft tissue with platelet concentrates of this magnitude.

Therefore, the working definition of effective PRP is a preparation that consists of more than 1,000,000 platelets/μl in a 5 ml volume of plasma. This forms a bioactive matrix or "gel" with active release of growth factors over 7 days.

Lesser platelet concentrations or non-viable platelets don't enhance wound healing. This means that the preparation of the platelet-rich plasma is critical.

Platelet gels and fibrin glues are effective agents for the prevention of further bleeding. At the same time, the platelets which participate in clot formation contain large reservoirs of proteins that participate in the healing and growth process. These proteins initiate and accelerate tissue repair and regeneration at the wound site.

To sum up the function of a clot:

- It acts as a hemostatic sealant/barrier
- It serves as a temporary scaffold to begin tissue regeneration
- It provides a location where growth factors can be concentrated
- It is also a location where stem cells can be attracted
- It provides a structure to which stem cells can bind

The platelet membrane has binding sites which attract T cells, B cells, and other white cell groups.

Undifferentiated cells are recruited to a site of injury through a process of chemo-attraction and migration.

Also, mitosis (division and multiplication) of undifferentiated cells occurs leading to larger numbers of cells.

Platelet growth factors also bind to receptors on the surface of stem cells leading to further division and multiplication of any stem cells located in the area.

A good PRP system will have the following characteristics:

- It will concentrate platelets to a level of roughly 5 to 7 times over baseline platelet counts
- The concentrated platelets will be viable
- When activated, the platelets will be able to release their growth factors over the next 7-10 days

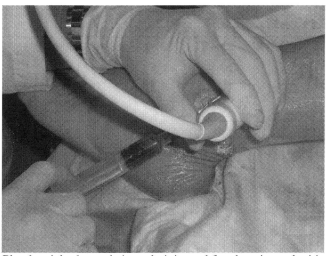

Platelet-rich plasma being administered for chronic tendonitis of the peroneal tendon using ultrasound guidance.

# Chapter 4

# Doctor... Tell Me About Platelet-Rich Plasma For Tendonitis And Arthritis...

The holy grail in arthritis and tendonitis treatment is to institute treatments that help regenerate normal tissue in areas where there has been damage due to injury or wear and tear. Research into the use of stem cells for this purpose looks promising.

To date, one area where accelerated tissue healing has been demonstrated is wound healing with the use of platelet-rich plasma. As it turns out, this substance is now being used to help accelerate the healing of conditions such as tendonitis, ligament strains, muscle strains, arthritis, synovitis (inflammation inside the joint), and cartilage defects.

Platelet-rich plasma is employed as a matrix graft, often referred to as an autologous tissue graft. This platelet-rich plasma (PRP) matrix is defined as a "tissue graft incorporating autologous growth factors and/or autologous undifferentiated cells in a cellular matrix where design depends on the receptor site and tissue of regeneration." (Crane D, Everts PAM. Practical Pain Management. 2008; January/February: 12- 26, 2008)

PRP is a normal blood clot with a much higher concentration of platelets (5 to 7 times).

Platelets make up about 6 percent of whole blood. Platelets make up 94 percent of a PRP specimen.

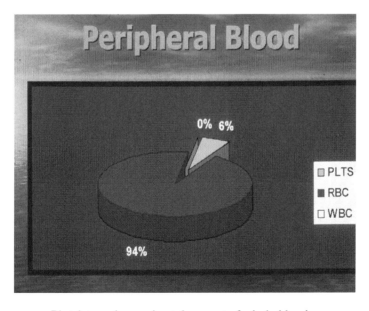

Platelets make up about 6 percent of whole blood

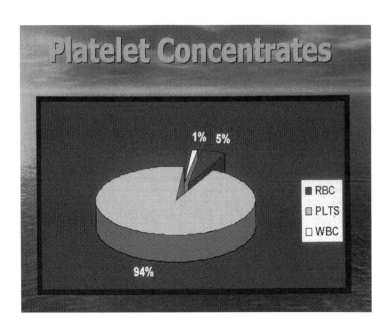

A PRP specimen contains 94 percent platelets

The reason this substance is so useful is that platelets, which are a constituent of normal blood, contain multiple growth factors that stimulate tissue growth. This is particularly true for collagen which is the main component of connective tissue such as tendons and cartilage. These factors include transforming growth factor-B (TGF-B), fibroblast growth factor, platelet-derived growth factor, epidermal growth factor, connective tissue growth factor, and vascular endothelial growth factor. In addition, PRP also has other vital to healing ingredients such as fibronectin, fibrin, and vitronectin.

These growth factors recruit undifferentiated cells to the site of injury and stimulate their growth. Another constituent of platelets, stromal cell derived factor I alpha, causes newly formed tissue to heal.

Normal healing goes through three distinct phases: inflammation, proliferation, and remodeling.

When we use PRP, we are actually trying to induce inflammation.

The inflammatory phase consists of the following activities:

- Bacterial killing
- Clotting
- Release of chemical messengers
- Release of growth factors
- Attraction of scavenger cells
- Start of the proliferative phase

During the inflammatory phase, the following occur:

- Platelets release
  - Coagulation factors
  - Platelet activating factors
  - Cytokines
  - Chemokines
- White blood cells and scavenger cells remove debris
- Blood flow is increased

Interestingly, during this phase, if there are stem cells in the vicinity, the various growth factors present in PRP will stimulate the stem cells to divide and multiply.

After the inflammatory phase, the proliferative phase begins (about 48-72 hours after the initial injury) and consists of:

- Fibroblast cells laying down collagen
- New blood vessels forming
- Shrinkage of the wound

This phase lasts 2-4 weeks.

The final phase is the remodeling phase:

- Blood vessels disappear
- New forms of collagen lead to increased tissue strength
- Tissue repair occurs

This phase can last a year.

This type of autologous tissue graft (ATG) is currently being used in musculoskeletal medicine for patients with pain and injury in joints, tendons, and ligaments.

Contrast this approach with the traditional approach which has been to use non-steroidal anti-inflammatory drugs as well as steroid injections, which, while reducing inflammation, also impede the healing process.

ATG is often used in conjunction with percutaneous tenotomy where a patient undergoes a procedure where there is purposeful needle irritation of the affected area using ultrasound guidance after which PRP is then slowly injected into the site.

The use of diagnostic ultrasound has revolutionized the field of musculoskeletal medicine. It facilitates tissue healing procedures like tenotomy which often prevent the need for open surgical procedures with their attendant morbidity and mortality.

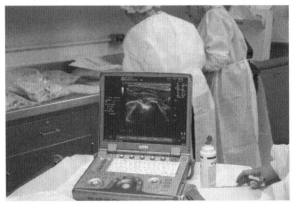
Ultrasound guidance is key

Sometimes, more than one treatment, perhaps two to three separated by four to eight week intervals are required.

The PRP is prepared by drawing 60 cc's of whole blood from the patient and then spinning the blood in a special centrifuge that layers out the platelets. This 60 cc's of whole blood generally yields about 2-10 cc's of platelet rich plasma.

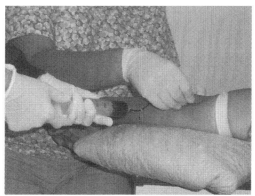
Drawing blood for PRP

Contraindications to the administration of PRP include platelet dysfunction, low platelet count, infection, and anemia.

Risks of PRP procedures include:

- 1:50,000 chance of introducing infection
- Allergy to anesthetic
- Pain of procedure
- Excessive bleeding
- Puncture of internal organ
- Injury as a result of procedure

Prior to a PRP procedure, patients need to hold their non-steroidal anti-inflammatory drugs for at least 3-4 days. They may resume them one week after. Also, patients with rheumatoid arthritis should hold their methotrexate for at least one week before and one week after the procedure... and sometimes longer. Patients on biologic medicines may need to hold their medicines longer, particularly when it comes to adalimumab (Humira), infliximab (Remicade), ocreluzimab (Simponi), and certolizumab (Cimzia) because of the long half life of these drugs. The reason again is that immunosuppressive and anti-inflammatory drugs impede wound healing.

Those taking low dose aspirin for heart prophylaxis may continue it. All other non-steroidal anti-inflammatory drugs, though, need to be discontinued.

Following the procedure, patients must rest the affected area to prevent leakage of the PRP from the site. The duration of rest will vary.

Pain at the injection site is common for a 1-2 day period following the procedure.

- The most intense pain lasts for 2-3 days, then slowly diminishes over 10 days
- There is a roller coaster of good and bad days

# Chapter 5

# What Types of Bursitis Are There?

In this chapter I'll talk about some of the more common types of bursitis. Let's start from the top and work down.

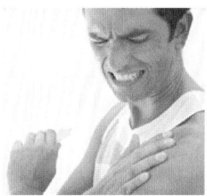
Shoulder pain often is due to bursitis

In the shoulder there is a large bursa called the subdeltoid bursa. This sits underneath the deltoid muscle which lies on the side of the upper arm at the shoulder. This is also called the subacromial bursa. Bursitis in this area presents with aching soreness in the shoulder that is aggravated by movement. Pain is present at night also. Over activity is the usual cause and it's common for rotator cuff tendonitis to coexist with this type of bursitis.

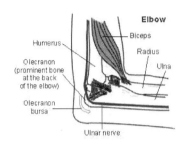

Olecrenon bursitis presents with swelling at
the tip of the elbow

The olecranon bursa is located at the tip of the elbow. Bursitis can develop as a result of excessive pressure (i.e. leaning on the elbow on a hard surface) or after significant trauma. One complication of this type of bursitis is that it can be become infected. The usual organism associated with septic bursitis is staph aureus. The treatment for septic bursitis is to drain the affected bursa and treat with antibiotics. Oral antibiotics usually work but intravenous antibiotics are sometimes needed.

The hip is an area where a number of different types of bursitis can occur. Prolonged sitting on a hard surface leads to ischiogluteal bursitis. This is a nagging type of bursitis located in the buttock region.

Iliopectineal bursitis is located in the groin area and is aggravated by walking, running, and going up stairs.

Trochanteric bursitis is located at the outside of the hip. This type of bursitis often occurs in overweight people and is aggravated by walking, going up stairs, and lying on the affected side.

Gluteus medius bursitis looks a lot like trochanteric bursitis. The location is usually a bit posterior to the trochanteric bursa.

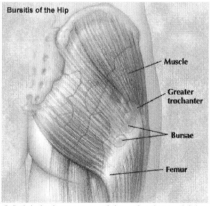

Multiple bursae cushion the lateral hip

Bursitis in the knee can be located either in front of the patella (prepatellar bursitis) or just below the knee along the inside of the upper part of the lower leg bone (tibia). This is called anserine bursitis. Prepatellar bursitis, as is the case with olecranon bursitis, can become septic.

Bursitis in the ankle can occur at the back of the heel beneath the Achilles tendon. Usually overactivity such as running too much can cause this type of bursitis. Rest, ice, and sometimes anti-inflammatory drugs are useful. Steroid injections should be used with great caution in this area because of the possibility of weakening the Achilles tendon. This situation can lead to rupture of the tendon.

Bursitis occurring at the base of the fifth toe is called a bunionette and bursitis occurring at the side of the large toe is called a bunion. Osteoarthritis is the usual underlying cause of the bursitis.

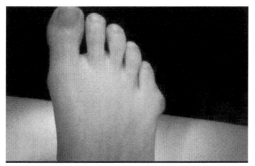

Bunionette

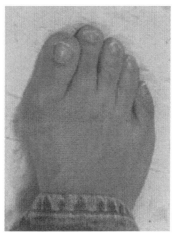

Bunion

Special padding and injections of glucocorticoids are helpful treatments.

Patients with inflammatory diseases such as gout or rheumatoid arthritis can also develop bursitis. Any patient with recurrent bursitis should be evaluated for an underlying condition that may be predisposing them to getting bursitis.

The diagnosis of bursitis and the treatment is not an easy one. A well-qualified rheumatologist or orthopedist should be consulted.

Conservative treatment measures include rest, stretching, ice, physical therapy, and glucocorticoid injection. If injection is required, ultrasound needle guidance is recommended.
For those who do not respond to these more conservative techniques, PRP is recommended.

# Chapter 6

# Amazing Shoulder Pain Reversing Secrets!

Whether you're a weekend athlete, or a gardener that overdid it, or a person with arthritis, there's hope for you. Shoulder problems are one of the most common afflictions of modern times. Fortunately, there are many ways of helping people feel better.

**The shoulder is the largest, most complex, and most mobile joint in the body**

Four muscles and their tendons (ropes attached to the top of the humerus), collectively known as the rotator cuff allow the shoulder to move as it does. The rotator cuff also plays a role in stabilizing the arm bone to the shoulder blade. In addition to the tendons and muscles of the rotator cuff, there are many other muscles and ligaments that lend stability to the shoulder. Plus, there is a rim of tissue that runs around the glenoid- the cup of the shoulder blade- that interacts with the humerus. This rim of tissue, called the glenoid labrum, provides more stability.

**Shoulder pain doesn't always come from the shoulder**

Examples include pain referred from arthritis of the neck, diseases of the chest such as pneumonia, and diseases of the abdomen like gallbladder problems can cause pain to be referred to the shoulder. Even ectopic pregnancies have caused shoulder pain!!!

Finally, heart conditions can cause referred pain to the shoulder, particularly on the left side. A specialist's physical exam is important.

I once saw a patient who had shoulder pain. The pupil of the eye on the same side of the shoulder was enlarged. That set off alarm bells so I ordered a chest x-ray. He turned out to have lung cancer. This combination is called Horner's syndrome.

**Most causes of true shoulder pain fall into 3 categories**

- Tendonitis/bursitis- With repetitive motion, the bursae (small fluid filled sacs) surrounding the shoulder joint can become inflamed. This condition is called bursitis.

- Injury/instability- Positions such as keeping your arms extended above your head will hurt the shoulder. Chronic compression, i.e. forcing the shoulder into its socket, due to injury, also is harmful. Finally, muscle imbalance- if one of the rotator cuff muscles is extra weak- can cause the rotator cuff to function poorly and lead to shoulder pain.
- Arthritis- Usually a function of aging.

**Patient tips:**

- Try to limit the number of overhead reaches.
- If you're wheelchair-bound, tuck your arms a bit closer to your body as you push.
- Avoid repetitive motion.
- Work on rotator cuff strengthening. Range-of-motion exercises are important!
- Use correct posture!

Oral anti-inflammatory medicines are sometimes, but not always, helpful. Patients may require a steroid injection.

For people who don't respond to medicines, injections, and physical therapy, another option is surgery. Any type of surgery should be done by a skilled shoulder surgeon. The shoulder is the most complex joint so make sure whoever works on your shoulder is an expert with shoulders.

One option to be considered...

Percutaneous needle tenotomy and platelet-rich plasma can stimulate the production of new strong tendon tissue.

# Chapter 7

# Platelet-Rich Plasma (PRP) For Achilles Tendonitis

The Achilles tendon is the largest tendon in the body and connects the gastrocnemius (calf muscle) to the back of the calcaneus (heel bone).

The Achilles tendon is what allows a person to stand up on their toes as well as jump up and down. The Achilles tendon is extremely strong and is capable of withstanding forces of 1,000 pounds or more.

However, it is also frequently predisposed to overuse and injury.

Achilles tendonitis causes localized pain which is often very severe in the tendon. Pain is usually felt about an inch and a half above the point where the Achilles tendon is attached to the heel. The pain is aggravated by running or by walking, particularly when the ambulation is uphill.

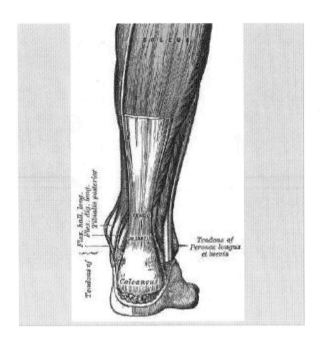

Achilles Tendon

The pain is typically aggravated by walking and relieved by rest.

While often occurring after exercise for which a person has either not warmed up for, or is unaccustomed to doing, Achilles tendonitis may also develop following direct injury. It may also present without a specific predisposing event.

Some forms of inflammatory arthritis such as psoriatic arthritis, Reiter's disease, and ankylosing spondylitis may cause Achilles inflammation. However, this type of inflammatory problem is distinct from the Achilles tendonitis occurring with overuse.

**www.arthritistreatmentcenter.com**

The typical conservative non surgical approach has been to use rest, non-steroidal anti-inflammatory drugs (NSAIDS), orthotics, stretching, massage, and therapeutic ultrasound.

Unfortunately, Achilles tendonitis may not respond to these measures. In the past, orthopedic surgeons would operate and the recuperative period would be lengthy.

However, a newer treatment for tendonitis may be more effective and prevent the need for surgery. Percutaneous needle tenotomy is a technique where a small gauge needle is introduced using local anesthetic with ultrasound guidance. The needle is used to poke several small holes in the tendon. This procedure is called "tenotomy."

The needle needs to be long enough to reach most areas of the Achilles. The procedure should not hurt if correct anesthetic procedures are used.

Tenotomy induces an acute inflammatory response. Then, platelet-rich plasma, obtained from a sample of the patient's whole blood is injected into the area where tenotomy has been performed. Platelets are cells that contain multiple healing and growth factors.

These include the following:

- Fibrinogen: helps with clotting and framework making
- Adhesion molecules: helps cells to bind to each other
- Platelets: initiates clotting and inflammation
- IL-1: promotes migration of macrophages
- Platelet derived growth factor: helps with healing; stimulates growth of blood vessels; attracts macrophages
- Transforming growth factor B: stimulates formation of collagen
- Epidermal growth factor: stimulates connective tissue growth
- Vascular endothelial growth factor: stimulates formation of new blood vessels; promotes healing

The result? Normal good quality fascial tissue is stimulated to grow with natural healing of the tendon. With severe tendonitis, a patient may need to wear a boot for 2 weeks following the procedure.

While most people respond to one course of treatment, about 10-20 percent of patients will require a second procedure.

Whether a second procedure is needed is usually determined at 4-6 weeks following the initial procedure. Diagnostic ultrasound using Doppler to assess the amount of residual inflammation is useful.

I underwent this very procedure in 2009. I was apprehensive, but it didn't hurt, and I can run again!

# Chapter 8

## Plantar Fasciitis... Heel Pain That Won't Go Away... What Can I Do?

Plantar fasciitis is one of the most common, painful foot problems. It is a syndrome where degeneration of the band of tissue that runs from the heel along the arch of the foot develops. Often, a heel spur accompanies the problem. Contrary to belief, the spur is the result of, and not the cause of the fasciitis.

Approximately, 70 percent of patients with plantar fasciitis have a heel spur that is visible on x-ray.

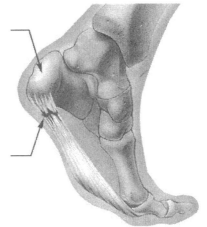

Plantar fasciitis

**www.arthritistreatmentcenter.com**

The plantar fascia is strong and thick and is responsible for maintaining the arch of the foot. Since it bears the brunt of weight on the foot with walking and running, it is the recipient of a tremendous amount of stress.

Plantar fasciitis occurs in two million Americans a year and 10 percent of the population over a lifetime. It is commonly associated with prolonged periods of weight-bearing. Obesity is a big risk factor.

Symptoms of plantar fasciitis are typically worse early in the morning after a night's sleep. When a patient arises, the pain in the bottom of the heel is excruciating… "Like an ice pick has been jammed into the heel." The pain subsides gradually with walking.

During the day, if a patient sits for any length of time, then gets up and walks again, the pain returns.

With a bit more walking, the pain soon decreases, only to return again with prolonged weight-bearing.

Treatment of plantar fasciitis involves the following:

Avoiding the inciting activity; As an example, a patient should take a few days off jogging or prolonged standing or walking. Resting usually helps to eliminate the pain, and will allow the discomfort to cool down.

Icing will help to reduce some of the symptoms and control the heel pain. Icing is especially helpful after an acute flare of symptoms.

Exercises and stretches are designed to relax the tissues that surround the heel bone. Some simple exercises, performed in the morning and evening, can help patients feel better quickly.

Anti-inflammatory medications help to relieve pain and decrease inflammation. Both over-the-counter and prescription options may be helpful.

Shoe inserts can lead to successful treatment of plantar fasciitis. The shoe inserts often permit patients to continue their routine activities without pain. They work by supporting the arch.

Night splints are worn to keep the heel stretched during sleep. By doing so, the arch of the foot does not contract at night, and is less painful in the morning.

If the pain does not resolve, the old approach was to administer a shot of cortisone to relieve inflammation.

However, there are potentially serious problems with cortisone injections. The two problems that can occur are fat pad atrophy and plantar fascial rupture. Both of these problems occur in a very small percentage of patients, but they can cause a worsening of heel pain symptoms.

A new treatment for chronic plantar fasciitis, called extracorporeal shock wave therapy, or ESWT, uses energy pulses to induce microtrauma to the tissue of the plantar fascia. This microtrauma is thought to induce tissue repair. Some people do well with this.

The treatment approach of choice though is percutaneous needle tenotomy with autologous tissue grafting. In this procedure, a physician will introduce a small needle under ultrasound guidance and use it to poke small holes in the plantar fascial attachment at the heel.

Following this, platelet-rich plasma, a concentrate of plasma from the patient's own blood is injected into the tenotomized area. The platelet-rich plasma contains abundant growth and healing factors. The plantar fascial tissue is regenerated.

In patients who do not respond to these measures, surgery is suggested.

# Chapter 9

# What is "PRP" and How Does it Work? Will it Help Me?

One exciting approach to wound healing, variously described as "regenerative medicine" or "tissue engineering" has been the use of platelet-rich plasma (PRP) either alone or in conjunction with stem cells.

PRP received notoriety when it was mentioned that Hines Ward, the Pittsburgh Steeler's star wide receiver had received this treatment for an injury prior to the Super Bowl.

Since then, many other athletes in the news have been treated with PRP, including Troy Polamalu, Dara Torres, and Tiger Woods.

As it turns out, PRP has been used for quite some time now, particularly at our center, to help accelerate the healing of conditions such as tendonitis, ligament strains, muscle strains, arthritis, synovitis (inflammation inside the joint), and cartilage defects.

Platelet-rich plasma is employed as a matrix graft, often referred to as an autologous tissue graft. This platelet-rich plasma (PRP) matrix is defined as a "Tissue graft incorporating autologous growth factors and/or autologous undifferentiated cells in a cellular matrix where design depends on the receptor site and tissue of regeneration." (Crane D, Everts PAM. Practical Pain Management. 2008; January/February: 12- 26) 2008)

The reason PRP is so useful is that platelets, which are a normal blood cell, contain multiple growth factors that stimulate tissue growth. In particular, PRP stimulates the growth of collagen which is the main component of connective tissue such as tendons and cartilage. These factors include transforming growth factor-B (TGF-B), fibroblast growth factor, platelet-derived growth factor, epidermal growth factor, connective tissue growth factor, and vascular endothelial growth factor.

These growth factors recruit undifferentiated cells to the site of injury and stimulate their growth. Another constituent of platelets, stromal cell derived factor I alpha causes newly recruited cells to adhere to the area.

In addition, when used with stem cells harvested from the patient's bone marrow, PRP "fires off" the stem cells to multiply quickly. This inflammatory response is what drives healing.

To use an analogy, PRP- particularly when used in conjunction with stem cells- sends the healing process into "warp drive."

PRP needs to be prepared in a way to ensure a maximal amount of platelets along with a high concentration of growth factors. Obviously, the more growth factors that can be delivered to the site of injury, the more likely tissue healing takes place.

This regenerative approach is diametrically opposite to the traditional method of healing tissue injuries which has been to use non-steroidal anti-inflammatory drugs as well as steroid injections, which, while reducing inflammation, also markedly impede the healing process.

PRP is often used in conjunction with percutaneous tenotomy. This is a procedure where there is purposeful needle irritation of the affected area using ultrasound guidance after which PRP is then slowly injected into the site.

The use of diagnostic ultrasound has revolutionized the field of musculoskeletal medicine in allowing tissue healing procedures like tenotomy which often prevent the need for open surgical procedures with their attendant morbidity and mortality. In the successful use of PRP and/or stem cells in tissue engineering, it is imperative that diagnostic ultrasound be used to guide the "needling" as well as the placement of the PRP.

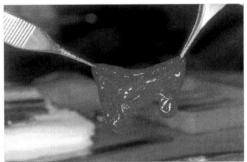

Clot typical for a good PRP preparation

The PRP is prepared by drawing 60 cc's of whole blood from the patient and then spinning the blood in a special centrifuge that layers out the platelets. This 60 cc's of whole blood generally yields about 2-10 cc's of platelet-rich plasma.

Contraindications to the administration of PRP include platelet dysfunction, low platelet count, infection, and anemia.

While one treatment works for the majority of patients, sometimes two to three treatments separated by four to eight week intervals may be required. The need for another treatment can be determined by using Doppler ultrasound to see if the area remains inflamed (good) or has gone "cold" (bad).

One caveat that bears repeating:

To reiterate, prior to a PRP procedure, a patient needs to hold their non-steroidal anti-inflammatory drugs for at least 3-4 days. They may resume them one week after. Also, patients with rheumatoid arthritis should hold their methotrexate for at least one week before and one week after the procedure. Patients on biologic medicines may need to hold their medicines longer, particularly when it comes to adalimumab (Humira), infliximab (Remicade), ocreluzimab (Simponi), and certiluzimab (Cimzia) because of the long half life of these drugs.

Following the procedure, patients must rest the affected area to prevent leakage of the PRP from the site.

Pain at the injection site is common for a 1-2 day period following the procedure.

# Chapter 10

# The 15 Absolute Critical Questions to Ask Before You Get (Platelet-Rich Plasma) PRP

There has been a lot written about platelet-rich plasma (PRP) recently. It's been in the news and has been on television. Hines Ward, a wide receiver for the Pittsburgh Steelers, and Dara Torres, the Olympic swimmer, both received PRP for chronic tendon injuries. This treatment allowed both of these superb athletes to compete way ahead of schedule.

PRP has become a very popular item to talk about when the discussion focuses on the best way to treat chronic… or even acute injuries in both world-class athletes as well as in weekend warriors. You, yourself, may be a person who has had a chronic tendon or ligament injury. You may have gone through the usual gamut of therapies including physical therapy, non-steroidal anti-inflammatory drugs, steroid injections, and so on.

This chapter is written for you- the person who may be contemplating PRP, or other direction.

I've prepared a question and answer guide to help you- the patient- find out about when, who, and how you should get your PRP.

1.  Is PRP good for every injury? The answer is no. For severe injuries where the tendon is completely torn or the ligament is completely disrupted, surgery is the answer. PRP is good for tendon and ligament injuries that are less severe. Strains and sprains.

2.  Is the physician board-certified? Board eligibility is not enough. All that means is that the doctor has gone through a training program. It doesn't mean that he or she has actually taken the board certification exam and passed it. Sometimes the physician doesn't take the exam because of fear... and sometimes they don't pass the exam. How comfortable would you feel getting a procedure done by a person who isn't board-certified?

3.  What should their specialty be? It should be in this order: rheumatology; physical medicine and rehabilitation (physiatry); orthopedics; pain management. The best is a

rheumatologist. They know joint and soft tissue disease and are usually much gentler than the other specialists. Sports medicine doctors are also very good.

4. What type of training should they have had? First of all, all procedures should be done using ultrasound guidance. If they don't use ultrasound to guide their injections, run away as fast as you can. Ultrasound allows precise targeting of the affected area. Who wants a blind injection? The chance of a blind injection working is very low. Second, they should have more than a weekend course under their belt. Ask them what type of certification they have. Who has trained them? At the risk of embarrassing this person, Dr. Tom Clark is the absolute best trainer in the world. If a person is Clark-trained, they are good. You should be blunt and grill the physician about their training credentials when it comes to PRP.

5. How many cases should they have done? Good results come with experience. Unless they've done at least 200 cases, you're a guinea pig.

6. What do they use to create the PRP? They should use machines from either Arteriocyte or Harvest. These are the two best machines available.

7. Who prepares the PRP? If they aren't experienced, watch out! Preparation of the PRP is very, very important to the success of the procedure.

8. How much time is there between drawing blood for the PRP and the actual procedure? This will vary, depending on whether a stem cell procedure is also being done at the same time. If it's only a PRP procedure and you have to wait more than 30 minutes, you won't get the best result. While PRP can sit for a bit of time, too long is bad.

9. Does the doctor fenestrate before injecting the PRP? What this means is this… the proper way to administer PRP is to "irritate" the area with a needle in preparation for the PRP. This fenestration should be done at least 50 times. If the PRP is just injected without fenestration, it won't work.

10. Will PRP work for arthritis? In cases where a patient is not a good candidate for lubricant therapy (viscosupplementation) or they have failed steroid injections, PRP might be helpful for pain relief. For unknown reasons, PRP is useful for pain relief in many patients with arthritis for whom other more conservative therapies have failed. PRP should not be done in patients

who have stage 4 joints (bone on bone) unless the patient absolutely refuses, or, is not a candidate for joint replacement.

11. When will PRP not work in tendon problems? When there is a complete tear, PRP by itself will not be effective. A stem cell treatment might be more effective. For instance, we've had patients with full thickness rotator cuff tears in the shoulder or gluteus minimus and gluteus medius tears in the hip not respond to PRP but who did respond to stem cell procedures.

12. How long before you know whether the PRP has worked? PRP is not an overnight miracle cure. It takes time. However, if a patient isn't noticeably better within 4-6 weeks, it's time to consider the following options: another PRP procedure; a stem cell procedure; surgery. It may take 2-3 PRP procedures for healing to occur. While expensive, it is much less expensive than surgery and the time off required for surgical recovery.

13. What kind of anesthetic is used? Local or regional block only.

14. What types of post-procedural activities should be avoided? Here is where the staff of the place where you

get your PRP procedure should be most useful. You should receive comprehensive, easy-to-understand instructions with a follow-up with the doctor within one to two weeks.

15. What's the cost? The cost will vary, depending on the skill and experience of the practitioner. Beware of bargain basement prices. It's not like getting a steal in Filene's basement!

# Chapter 11
# PRP: Hope or Hype?

Steelers wide receiver, Hines Ward, underwent a medical procedure using platelet-rich plasma- PRP- before the Super Bowl XLIII. It allowed him to play in this critical game.

Tory Polamalu, the Steeler's superlative defensive player also had it. And more recently, Tiger Woods underwent the same type of treatment.

But exactly what is PRP and how effective is it?

Platelet-rich plasma is prepared by drawing blood from a patient, then placing the blood in a centrifuge which spins the blood at high speed in order to separate the platelets from the red blood cells. The resulting small volume of fluid after the centrifugation process contains approximately 5-7 times the normal volume of platelets.

As mentioned earlier, platelets are cells that contain an enormous amount of healing and growth factors such as:

- Fibrinogen: helps with clotting and framework making
- Adhesion molecules: helps cells to bind to each other
- Platelets: initiates clotting and inflammation
- IL-1: promotes migration of macrophages
- Platelet derived growth factor: helps with healing, stimulates growth of blood vessels, attracts macrophages
- Transforming growth factor B: stimulates formation of collagen
- Epidermal growth factor: stimulates connective tissue growth
- Vascular endothelial growth factor: stimulates formation of new blood vessels, promotes healing

The platelet rich plasma is then injected under ultrasound guidance to ensure proper placement of the PRP.

Multiple studies have shown that PRP can accelerate healing of soft tissue injuries such as tendonitis, ligament tears, and related problems.

One study that demonstrated the effectiveness of PRP was performed in patients with chronic elbow tendonitis (Mishra A, Pavelko T. Am J Sports Med. 2006; 34: 1774-1778). The authors evaluated 140 patients with chronic elbow tendonitis and treated them conservatively with physical therapy. Twenty of the patients failed to respond and were randomized to receive either PRP injection (n=15) or bupivicaine (local anesthetic) injection. The bupivicaine group served as the control group.

Eight weeks after the treatment, the platelet-rich plasma patients noted 60 percent improvement in their visual analog pain scores versus 16 percent improvement in control patients. Sixty percent (3 of 5) of the control subjects withdrew or sought other treatments after the 8-week period, preventing further direct analysis. Therefore, only the patients treated with platelet-rich plasma were available for continued evaluation. At 6 months, the patients treated with platelet-rich plasma noted 81 percent improvement in their visual analog pain scores. At final follow-up (mean, 25.6 months; range, 12–38 months), the platelet-rich plasma patients reported 93 percent reduction in pain compared with before the treatment. The authors concluded that PRP significantly reduced pain and should be considered for use before attempting surgery.

**www.arthritistreatmentcenter.com**

While PRP has been used via a "blind" approach- just injecting it "where it hurts," it has become quite clear that precise placement of the PRP is essential for optimal results. That's why ultrasound guided placement of the PRP is crucial. Actually… it's mandatory!

As far as Hines Ward, he had a sprain of the medial collateral ligament of the knee. While surgery could have been an option, it was decided to use PRP instead.

PRP can speed the rate of healing by about 50 percent.

Another innovation has been the use of stem cells in concert with PRP. We have had excellent results in treating a wide spectrum of disorders. While most cases of chronic tendonitis or bursitis will respond to PRP only, significant tendon injuries and conditions such as osteoarthritis require the use of stem cells along with the PRP.

After examining the patient and evaluating MRI results, we can decide which option- PRP alone or PRP with stem cells will work better for the patient. For accelerated healing only, PRP is fine. For healing plus tissue regeneration, stem cells should be added.

**www.arthritistreatmentcenter.com**

Stem cells are cells that haven't yet differentiated into a specific type of tissue. They can be stimulated to differentiate into any type of tissue needed provided the correct environment is arranged. In other words, if you place stem cells with heart cells, they become heart cells... if you place them with lung cells, they become lung cells. So if you place the stem cells near tendon or cartilage cells, you get tendon or cartilage.

We use autologous stem cells. These are the patient's own cells that we harvest from bone marrow obtained from the iliac crest of the hip. By using a patient's own cells, we don't run the risk of rejection reactions which you can get with stem cells from donors or unregulated growth which is theoretically possible with embryonic stem cells.

By customizing the treatment approach- using either PRP or PRP plus stem cells, depending on the situation- and using ultrasound needle guidance, we have had enormous success with accelerating tissue healing and tissue regrowth.

# Chapter 12

## Tell me more about PRP?

If an internet search is done, new information on platelet-rich plasma (PRP) is found on a daily basis. In the orthopedic and rheumatology literature there is intense debate over whether PRP actually works. Even now, there are many practitioners that remain skeptical regarding the effectiveness of this therapy.

To counterbalance this cynicism, there are some practitioners who have literally gone overboard to defend the use (and sometimes, abuse) of PRP. They wax enthusiastically about its many benefits and tout its effectiveness to the point that it has assumed the same significance as holy water.

The truth is probably somewhere in between.

What is certain is this…

PRP has been used extensively in Europe for years to treat tendonopathy (tendonitis) and other non-healing soft tissue injuries such as ligament tears.

The basic science suggests that platelets become activated after injection into tendons or soft tissue. Platelets used for the procedure are autologous, meaning they are derived from the patient. Whole blood is then centrifuged and platelets are separated from the remaining blood components and isolated in a specific chamber.

Once harvested, the platelets are injected into diseased tissue under ultrasound guidance so that the injecting needle is inserted exactly into the area of pathology.

Once injected, the platelets undergo activation and release numerous growth factors into the damaged and diseased area. These growth factors also recruit stem cells and other proteins that create new, healthy tissue.

PRP is used to treat tendon disorders such as rotator cuff tendonitis, lateral epicondylitis "tennis elbow," patellar tendonitis "jumper's knee," Achilles tendonitis, and many other conditions that are characterized by non-healing tissue.

PRP can also be used to treat partial tears of many tendons, ligaments, and muscles. It is often used to speed healing.

PRP injections are usually given as a series of one to three injections over a period of eight to twelve weeks.

PRP does not provide the instant pain relief that a corticosteroid ("cortisone") injection might. However, unlike corticosteroid, PRP leads to healing of previously unhealthy tissue. There is abundant evidence that corticosteroids, while helping with short term pain, actually have a deleterious effect on wound healing.

Prior to the PRP injection the diseased tendon(s) are usually fenestrated (multiple small holes are made with a needle) to increase blood flow to the area, provide channels for the PRP, and also to free up diseased tissue from arthritis spurs. The technical term for this is "tenotomy."

The overall success rate of PRP varies from practitioner to practitioner but should be in the 80 percent range. Success with PRP is highly dependent on the PRP preparation as well as the skill of the physician administering the procedure. Poorer outcomes occur in smokers, diabetics, and patients with compromised microcirculation, and patients on any type of immunosuppressive therapy.

As has been mentioned previously, patients who take anti-inflammatory drugs or immunosuppressive drugs as well as fish oil must hold these medications for a significant length of time both before as well as after the procedure.

Patients with rheumatoid arthritis who take methotrexate and biologics are especially hard to treat because of the time period required for them to hold their medication.

# Chapter 13

## Does PRP Really Work?

There has been much debate about the beneficial effects of platelet-rich plasma (PRP). While a Dutch study stated that PRP was no better than "placebo" for the treatment of chronic Achilles tendonitis, the "placebo" was a standard tenotomy protocol which is an effective therapy. So the fact that PRP was only a little better than an effective therapy doesn't say that PRP is not effective.

What was neglected by much of the media was the technique used to administer the PRP- not a technique that is favored by those of us who use PRP a lot. And the type of method used to prepare the PRP. Unless the protocol definitely produced a platelet concentration 4-5 times baseline, the treatment was not going to be effective.

Also, another more recent Dutch study did show PRP was very effective for lateral epicondylitis (tennis elbow) and an Italian study showed favorable results in osteoarthritis of the knee.

So… if you're a prospective patient with a tendonitis problem, how do you ensure you get the right type of treatment?

First, make sure the physician who administers the PRP has done at least 200 cases.

Second, make sure the physician is skilled in the use of diagnostic ultrasound.  Unless ultrasound is used, the PRP is essentially wasted.

Third, what type of protocol is used?  Find out the exact machine used and what the platelet concentration above baseline is administered.  It must be at least 4-5 times above baseline.

Fourth, make sure you don't have any of the conditions that might make a PRP procedure less than effective.  These include:

- Anti-platelet / anti-inflammatory medication
    - Coumadin, ASA, NSAIDS, heparin, etc…
    - High dose fish oil
- Bleeding/clotting disorder
- Anemia/low platelet count
- Cigarette smoking
- Nutritional/hormonal deficiency
- Diabetes

Here is a list of potential areas where PRP has been shown to be effective. This list is provided courtesy of Dr. Jonathan Fenton.

Hip/Pelvis

- Hip osteoarthritis
- Hamstring origin/ischial tuberosity tendinosis
- Symphysis pubis / pubalgia
- Adductor /gluteal tendinosis

Knee

- Patellar tendinosis
- Quadriceps tendinosis and tears
- Collateral/cruciate ligament tears
- Meniscal tears

- Osteoarthritis
- Patellofemoral osteoarthritis
- Post anterior cruciate ligament tears
- Pes anserine bursitis / tendinosis
- Proximal tibia-fibula joint laxity with osteoarthritis

Ankle/Foot

- Achilles tendinosis
- Peroneal tendinosis and tear
- Tibialis posterior tears and tendinosis
- Plantar fasciitis
- Osteochondral defect talus
- Sinus tarsi syndrome
- Ankle ligament tears and laxity
- Bunions
- Osteoarthritis ankle, foot, toes

And this is only a partial list.

When PRP is given it should be done after a percutaneous needle tenotomy is performed. This is a procedure where the damaged or diseased tendon is peppered with multiple small holes using ultrasound guidance. Why?

The procedure helps to break up scar tissue, abnormal blood vessels, and degenerative tissue. It also stimulates bleeding and creates a favorable condition for PRP.

Tenotomy also leads to remodeling of tendon in a way that restores many of its normal mechanical properties.
At the Arthritis Treatment Center, we have had enormous success using PRP for the above areas and highly recommend it for patients in whom chronic tendonitis is a problem.

# Chapter 14

# What kinds of problems can PRP solve?

There is controversy among both manufacturers of cell centrifuges as well as among practitioners who use platelet-rich plasma concentrates as to what constitutes a sufficient number of platelets.

A number of studies have hinted that the platelet concentrate and vascular endothelial growth factors within platelet concentrates stimulate mesenchymal stem cell multiplication in a dose dependent manner. In other words, the more platelets, the more stem cells are attracted to the area, and the more rapid the healing process.

To reiterate the sequence of events in healing from previous chapters…

First there is injury… then there is clot formation … then inflammation… then tissue regeneration… then tissue remodeling. The first three steps involve proteins found in the three major cell types found in circulating blood… white blood cells, red blood cells, and platelets.

The major working theory regarding the use of platelet concentrates has been this: Delivering a high concentration of tissue healing proteins to the site of injury may speed the rate of healing.

So what types of conditions respond to platelet rich plasma? We've already discussed a partial list submitted by Dr. Jonathan Fenton in an earlier chapter.

Here's another list of specific conditions, courtesy of the "Crane Clinic Sports Medicine" (Chesterfield, MO) and Riverside Sports, Spine, and Fitness Center (Riverside, OH)] include:

- Spine
- Sacroiliac joints
- Iliolumbar ligaments
- Facet joints
- Costotransverse (rib) joints

**www.arthritistreatmentcenter.com**

- Spinal ligaments

Shoulder

- Rotator cuff tendinosis/tears
- Biceps tendinosis
- Chronic glenohumeral ligament strains
- Shoulder joint arthritis
- Labral tears and degeneration

Elbows

- Epicondylitis (medial and lateral)
- Ulnar collateral ligament
- Distal biceps tendon
- Osteoarthritis

Wrist/Hand

- Chronic ulnar collateral ligament injury of thumb
- Osteoarthritis of the base of the thumb
- Tendinosis
- Osteoarthritis

Hip/Pelvis

- Hip osteoarthritis

**www.arthritistreatmentcenter.com**

- Hamstring origin
- Symphysis pubis
- Adductor/gluteal tendinosis

Knee

- Patellar tendinosis
- Quadriceps tendinosis and tears
- Collateral / cruciate ligament tears
- Meniscal tears
- Osteoarthritis
- Patellofemoral osteoarthritis
- Following anterior cruciate ligament repair
- Pes anserine bursitis / semitendinosis
- Proximal tibial-fibular joint laxity / osteoarthritis

Ankle/Foot

- Achilles tendinosis
- Peroneal tendinosis and tear
- Tibialis posterior tendon tears and tendinosis
- Plantar fasciitis
- Sinus tarsi syndrome
- Ankle ligament tears and laxity

**www.arthritistreatmentcenter.com**

- Bunions

What other studies do we have to show the effectiveness of PRP?

Mishra A, Pafelko T, Coetzee; "Treatment of Chronic Severe Elbow Tendinosis with PRP." *American Journal of Sports Medicine,* 34:1774-1778, 2006

Study: Twenty patients that failed non-operative treatment for chronic epicondylar pain were randomized to evaluate effectiveness of PRP – at one, two, and six months all PRP patients had lower pain and greater range of motion than control (bupivicaine). Treatment of chronic epicondylar pain with PRP should be considered prior to surgical intervention.

Sanchez M, et al; "Application of Autologous Growth Factors on Skeletal Muscle Healing." *World Congress on Regenerative Medicine Podium Presentation,* May 18, 2005

Study: Twenty patient prospective muscle injury pilot study with six month follow-up – Ultrasound guided injection of PRP within the injured muscle enhanced healing (echo-graphic images) and functional capacities 50 percent faster than the control group.

Barrett S, Erredge S; "Growth Factors for Chronic Plantar Fasciitis", *Podiatry Today,* 37-42, 2004

Study: Nine patients with hypoechoic and thickened plantar fascia were injected with PRP to evaluate the efficacy of PRP with one week, two week and one, three, six, and twelve month follow-up – All patients had improvement that was noted on diagnostic ultrasound and six patients had complete resolution after two months. At one year, seven of nine patients were completely healed.

The results from PRP are highly dependent on two major factors.

The first is the experience of the practitioner and the second is the use of ultrasound guidance to carry out the needed procedure.

The other major tool that separates the "pro" from the amateur is the ability to perform percutaneous needle tenotomy (PNT) using ultrasound guidance. Here's what's done...

- Debride/fenestrate -poke holes- in the tendon with needle (18-22g) under ultrasound guidance
- Breaks up scar tissue, and myxoid (gelatinous) degeneration; stimulates bleeding; creates favorable condition for PRP
- Leads to remodeling of tendon in a way that restores many of its normal mechanical properties
- Target any enthesophytes (bone spurs) by removing them with the cutting edge of the needle. This is called needle barbitage
- Perform an in-plane needle tenotomy meaning the tenotomy is performed along the long axis of the tendon fibers, not crosswise
- Instill the PRP in layers
- Fill in any defects in the cortex and tendon
- Mix with lidocaine
  - Using 2 percent lidocaine is better since there is lower dilution of PRP
  - Avoid long acting local anesthetics since they are toxic to muscle tissue and cartilage

- Always needle and inject the proximal and distal insertions of the tendon
  - Site of the most blood supply
- Inject the tear, if present
- Inject in a layered approach, along the long axis of the ligament, when possible
- If working inside a joint, avoid high concentrations of local anesthetics
- High doses of lidocaine are toxic to cartilage
- For muscle tears
  - Instill the PRP in layers into the muscle defect
  - In the long axis of the fibers, not across
  - Multiple needle passes
  - Post-injection bruising very common
- For joints
  - Aspirate effusions (joint fluid) if present
  - After waiting for adequate anesthesia, inject PRP
  - Then consider injecting with calcium chloride and thrombin
  - Generally repeat the three aforementioned steps at 4-8 week intervals
    - Two to three treatments for hips

**www.arthritistreatmentcenter.com**

- Three to five for knees
- Non-weight bearing for a minimum of 48 hours
- Try to pepper the defect gently
- Fill all areas of cartilage irregularity
- If the direct visualization of the defect is not possible, filling the joint itself will often do as well
  - May take more sessions
- Recommend activating intra-articular PRP with calcium chloride and thrombin
- PRP causes initial increase volume of fluid in the joint
  - Can be severe
  - Usually increased volume lasts three to seven days
  - Rarely have to remove fluid

In the experience of some practitioners, PRP can resolve joint fluid and joint inflammation. Obviously, more controlled studies are needed to confirm this.

# Conclusion

While much is known about the science of platelet-rich plasma, very few double-blind controlled studies have been done.

While the theory is extremely attractive, more research needs to be conducted before this type of treatment enters the mainstream.

We need to know what types of problems PRP will solve, what problems it won't solve, and what the options are.

Judging from the veterinary data as well as the anecdotal information available from athletes, PRP is a step in the right direction.

It may well be, along with stem cell therapy, the key to true regenerative medicine for musculoskeletal problems.

The final point is that PRP is as natural as you can get as far as a treatment. It's basically your own blood. The appeal is obvious.

The key point is this: should you decide to seek out a practitioner for PRP, use this book as your guide to finding the right expert.

I wish you the best of luck and good healing!

For more information on PRP, contact us at:

**Arthritis Treatment Center**
**71 Thomas Johnson Drive**
**Frederick, Maryland 21702**
**(301) 694-5800**
**(301) 694-0187 Fax**
**www.arthritistreatmentcenter.com**

**You may email me at:**
**nwei@arthritistreatmentcenter.com**

If you want to know more about PRP, go to
http://thebookonprp.com/prpbookoffer/ (password: prp) for the
ultimate consumer's guide on how to banish tendonitis:

You'll discover…

- How PRP helped win the Superbowl… and how it can
  help you win your battle against chronic tendonitis,
- The 6 major risks of PRP procedures… knowing them
  could save your life!
- The must have technique that makes a PRP procedure
  virtually painless,
- The 15 critical questions you need the answers to before
  you get PRP,
- Heal stubborn tendon tears with nature's "superglue."

You'll get 20% off the regular price of "How to Banish
Tendonitis – A Consumer's Guide to the Most Effective
Treatments."

Copy the following link on to your internet browser to take
advantage of these incredible savings and how PRP therapy may
help you!

http://thebookonprp.com/prpbookoffer/ (password: prp)

Made in the USA
Coppell, TX
26 April 2022

77062546R00055

Nathan Wei, MD is a graduate of Swarthmore College and the Jefferson Medical College. He completed his residency at the University of Michigan Medical Center in Ann Arbor, Michigan and his fellowship in arthritis at the National Institutes of Health in Bethesda, Maryland. Dr. Wei is an acknowledged national expert in rheumatoid arthritis and osteoarthritis and is the author of more than 500 publications. He is a Fellow of the American College of Physicians, a Fellow of the American College of Rheumatology, and is the only American rheumatologist member in the Arthroscopy Association of North America. Dr. Wei is considered an authority and expert in stem cell and platelet-rich plasma (PRP) procedures. He is active in clinical research and is the Director of the Arthritis Treatment Center, located in Frederick, Maryland.

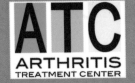

ATC
ARTHRITIS
TREATMENT CENTER

ISBN 9781453635452

90000

9 781453 635452